Gout-Friendly

Cookbook

Elevate Your Plate: A Flavorful Odyssey To Gout-Free

Living

STEVE OPERA

Copyright © 2023

All Rights Are Reserved

The content in this book may not be reproduced, duplicated, or transferred without the express written permission of the author or publisher. Under no circumstances will the publisher or author be held liable or legally responsible for any losses, expenditures, or damages incurred directly or indirectly as a consequence of the information included in this book.

Legal Remarks

Copyright protection applies to this publication. It is only intended for personal use. No piece of this work may be modified, distributed, sold, quoted, or paraphrased without the author's or publisher's consent.

Disclaimer Statement

Please keep in mind that the contents of this booklet are meant for educational and recreational purposes. Every effort has been made to offer accurate, up-to-date, reliable, and thorough information. There are, however, no stated or implied assurances of any kind. Readers understand that the author is providing competent counsel. The content in this book originates from several sources. Please seek the opinion of a competent professional before using any of the tactics outlined in this book. By reading this book, the reader agrees that the author will not be held accountable for any direct or indirect damages resulting from the use of the information contained therein, including, but not limited to, errors, omissions, or inaccuracies.

TABLE OF CONTENTS

INTRODUCTION

Understanding Gout

In this section, the book delves into an explanation of what gout is. It may cover aspects such as the causes, symptoms, and triggers of gout. The goal is to provide the reader with a comprehensive understanding of this medical condition.

Importance of a Gout-Friendly Diet

This part emphasizes the connection between diet and gout. It discusses how certain foods can contribute to the development or exacerbation of gout symptoms. It may also highlight the significance of making dietary choices that are conducive to managing and preventing gout attacks.

How This Cookbook Can Help

This section explains the purpose and benefits of the cookbook. It could include information on how the recipes and guidelines provided in the book are specifically designed to be gout-friendly. This may involve insights into ingredient choices, cooking methods, and overall meal planning strategies to support individuals in managing their gout through diet. It serves as an introduction to the practical aspects of the cookbook and sets the stage for what the reader can expect to gain from using it.

CHAPTER ONE

GOUT AND NUTRITION

Foods to Avoid with Gout

1. Organ meats (liver, kidneys, etc.)
2. Red meat (beef, lamb, pork)
3. Seafood high in purines (anchovies, sardines, mackerel)
4. Shellfish (shrimp, crab, lobster)
5. Game meats (venison, duck, goose)
6. Gravy and meat-based sauces
7. High-fructose corn syrup (found in many processed foods)
8. Sugary beverages
9. Alcohol, especially beer and spirits
10. Processed and cured meats (bacon, sausage, hot dogs)
11. High-fat dairy products
12. Fried foods
13. White bread and refined carbohydrates
14. Asparagus
15. Spinach
16. Cauliflower
17. Mushrooms

18. Lentils

19. Beans (especially kidney beans)

20. Peas

21. Oatmeal

22. Whole grain products in excess

23. Yeast-based products (bread, beer)

24. Fatty fish (salmon, trout)

25. Sweetbreads

26. Mussels

27. Scallops

28. Caviar

29. Beer

30. Anchovies

31. Herring

32. Trout

33. Tuna

34. Sweetened cereals

35. Sugary snacks and desserts

36. High-fat snacks (chips, fries)

37. Processed foods with high sodium content

38. High-fat gravies

39. Game meats (venison, rabbit)

40. Consommé

41. Bouillon

42. Gelatin desserts made with organ meats

43. Wild game

44. Sweetened fruit juices

45. Sugary jams and jellies

46. Excessive coffee consumption

47. Excessive tea consumption

48. High-purine vegetables (asparagus, cauliflower, spinach)

49. Excessive consumption of vitamin C supplements

50. High-fat sauces and dressings

Gout-Triggering Ingredients

1. High-fructose corn syrup

2. Added sugars

3. Artificial sweeteners

4. Alcohol

5. Yeast extracts

6. Monosodium glutamate (MSG)

7. Soy sauce

8. Highly processed foods

9. Saturated fats

10. Trans fats

11. Hydrogenated oils

12. Fried foods

13. Processed meats

14. Shellfish

15. Organ meats

16. Red meat

17. Processed poultry

18. Bacon

19. Sausages

20. Hot dogs

21. High-purine vegetables (asparagus, spinach)

22. Cauliflower

23. Mushrooms

24. Beans (especially kidney beans)

25. Lentils

26. Peas

27. Oatmeal

28. Whole grain products in excess

29. White bread

30. Refined carbohydrates

31. High-fat dairy

32. Full-fat yogurt

33. Ice cream

34. Certain nuts (like peanuts)

35. Certain seeds (like sunflower seeds)

36. Sardines

37. Anchovies

38. Trout

39. Tuna

40. Scallops

41. Mussels

42. Caviar

43. Sweetbreads

44. Game meats (venison, rabbit)

45. Fatty fish (salmon, trout)

46. Beer

47. Spirits

48. Sweetened fruit juices

49. Excessive coffee

50. Excessive tea

Nutritional Guidelines for Gout Management

Managing gout through proper nutrition involves making informed choices to control uric acid levels and reduce the risk of painful flare-ups. Here are key nutritional guidelines for individuals with gout:

Hydration is Key:

Ensure adequate water intake to help flush out uric acid from the body. Aim for at least 8 glasses (64 ounces) of water per day.

Balance Your Diet:

Strive for a well-balanced diet that includes a variety of fruits, vegetables, whole grains, lean proteins, and low-fat dairy. This can help maintain a healthy weight and support overall well-being.

Moderate Protein Intake:

Choose lean protein sources such as poultry, fish, tofu, and legumes. Limit red meat, organ meats, and seafood high in purines, which can contribute to uric acid buildup.

Limit Purine-Rich Foods:

Minimize consumption of high-purine foods, including organ meats, certain seafood, and some vegetables like asparagus and spinach.

Healthy Fats:

Opt for healthy fats found in olive oil, avocados, and nuts. Avoid saturated and trans fats commonly found in processed foods and fried items.

Moderate Alcohol Consumption:

Limit alcohol intake, particularly beer and spirits, as they can elevate uric acid levels. Moderate wine consumption may be a more gout-friendly option for some.

Control Portion Sizes:

Practice portion control to manage calorie intake and maintain a healthy weight. Overeating, especially of high-calorie foods, can contribute to gout symptoms.

Choose Low-Fat Dairy:

Include low-fat or fat-free dairy products in your diet. These can provide essential nutrients without contributing to excessive purine levels.

Limit Added Sugars:

Reduce the consumption of sugary foods and beverages, as they may contribute to weight gain and increase the risk of gout attacks.

Monitor Fructose Intake:

Be mindful of fructose from sources like sweetened beverages and certain fruits, as excessive fructose intake may impact uric acid levels.

Moderate Caffeine Intake:

While coffee consumption in moderation is generally considered safe, excessive caffeine intake should be avoided as it may affect uric acid levels for some individuals.

Consider Vitamin C:

Some studies suggest that vitamin C may help lower uric acid levels. Include vitamin C-rich foods such as citrus fruits, strawberries, and bell peppers in your diet.

CHAPTER TWO

BUILDING GOUT-FRIENDLY MEALS

Balancing Flavors and Textures

Achieving a harmonious blend of flavors and textures is a culinary art that enhances the enjoyment of meals while adhering to gout-friendly principles. This section explores the importance of balancing taste profiles, including savory, sweet, sour, and umami, to create well-rounded dishes. Additionally, attention is given to the interplay of textures, such as incorporating crispiness, creaminess, and tenderness, to elevate the overall dining experience.

Key Considerations:

Savoring Savory:

Explore the use of herbs, spices, and low-purine umami-rich ingredients to enhance the savory dimension of dishes without relying on high-purine sources.

Subtle Sweetness:

Incorporate natural sweetness from fruits and select vegetables to add a pleasing sweetness to dishes, avoiding excessive sugars and fructose.

Tangy Twists:

Introduce acidity through citrus fruits, vinegar, or low-purine sources to bring a refreshing tanginess that complements other flavors.

Umami Magic:

Embrace umami-rich ingredients like mushrooms, tomatoes, and certain cheeses to impart depth and richness without compromising gout-friendly principles.

Crunchy Contrasts:

Integrate textures like nuts, seeds, or crisp vegetables to provide a satisfying crunch, adding a dynamic element to the overall culinary experience.

Creamy Indulgences:

Utilize low-fat dairy or alternative sources to achieve creaminess in dishes without elevating saturated fats, contributing to a healthier balance.

Tender Delicacies:

Explore cooking techniques that result in tender and succulent proteins, ensuring a satisfying texture without relying on high-purine options.

Experimenting with Combinations:

Encourage culinary creativity by experimenting with combinations of flavors and textures, keeping in mind the principles of a gout-friendly diet.

Portion Control and Gout

Effective portion control plays a pivotal role in managing gout and promoting overall well-being. This section focuses on the importance of mindful eating habits and maintaining appropriate serving sizes to mitigate the risk of gout flare-ups and support a healthy lifestyle.

Key Points:

Preventing Overconsumption:

Discuss the impact of excessive food intake, especially high-purine foods, on uric acid levels and the potential for triggering gout attacks. Emphasize the need to avoid overindulgence to maintain a balanced diet.

Understanding Serving Sizes:

Provide practical guidance on recognizing appropriate portion sizes for various food groups, emphasizing the importance of moderation to prevent excessive calorie and purine intake.

Balancing Nutrient Intake:

Encourage individuals to focus on a balanced distribution of nutrients in each meal, ensuring that portions of proteins, carbohydrates, and fats align with dietary recommendations for gout management.

Listening to Hunger Cues:

Advocate for mindful eating by paying attention to hunger and fullness cues. Understanding one's body signals helps prevent overeating and supports maintaining a healthy weight.

Strategies for Smaller Portions:

Offer tips on reducing portion sizes without sacrificing satisfaction, such as using smaller plates, sharing meals, and savoring each bite mindfully.

Smart Snacking:

Discuss the importance of portion control in snacks, suggesting gout-friendly options and providing ideas for satisfying small bites between meals.

Avoiding Second Helpings:

Highlight the potential risks associated with going back for seconds, especially with foods that may contribute to gout symptoms, and encourage restraint.

Building Awareness:

Promote a heightened awareness of portion sizes when dining out or enjoying pre-packaged foods, as these may often contain larger servings than necessary.

Personalized Approaches:

Acknowledge that individual nutritional needs vary, and recommend consulting with healthcare professionals or dietitians to tailor portion control strategies to specific health conditions and goals.

Creating Satisfying Gout-Friendly Menus

Crafting menus that are both delicious and aligned with gout management principles requires thoughtful planning and creativity. This section provides practical insights and tips on how to design satisfying menus that cater to the unique dietary needs of individuals with gout.

Key Strategies:

Diverse Protein Sources:

Explore a variety of lean protein options such as poultry, fish, tofu, and legumes to ensure a good balance without relying heavily on high-purine choices.

Abundant Vegetables:

Incorporate a colorful array of vegetables, focusing on those with lower purine content. This not only adds nutritional value but also contributes to satisfying and visually appealing meals.

Whole Grains for Sustenance:

Choose whole grains like quinoa, brown rice, and oats to provide sustained energy and dietary fiber, promoting a feeling of fullness without compromising gout-friendly principles.

Mindful Portioning:

Implement portion control strategies to prevent overconsumption, offering satisfying meals without exceeding recommended calorie or purine limits.

Flavorful Herbs and Spices:

Enhance the taste of dishes with flavorful herbs and spices, allowing for the creation of tasty meals without relying on excessive salt, sugar, or high-purine seasonings.

Balanced Meals:

Design menus that include a balance of macronutrients – proteins, carbohydrates, and fats – to meet nutritional needs while adhering to gout management guidelines.

Creative Culinary Techniques:

Explore cooking methods that add depth and richness to dishes without compromising health, such as grilling, roasting, or using healthy fats for flavor.

Hydration with Flair:

Incorporate hydrating options like infused water, herbal teas, and low-sugar beverages to complement meals and enhance the overall dining experience.

Variety in Meal Types:

Provide ideas for diverse meals, including breakfast, lunch, dinner, and snacks, ensuring that individuals with gout can enjoy a satisfying range of flavors and textures throughout the day.

Adapting Favorite Recipes:

Guide readers on modifying their favorite recipes to be gout-friendly, encouraging flexibility in culinary choices while adhering to dietary recommendations.

Seasonal and Local Ingredients:

Promote the use of seasonal and locally sourced ingredients to maximize freshness and flavor, contributing to the overall appeal of gout-friendly menus.

CHAPTER THREE

GOUT-FRIENDLY COOKING TECHNIQUES

Low-Purine Cooking Methods

When preparing meals for gout management, choosing cooking methods that minimize the release of purines is essential. Here are cooking techniques that help retain flavor and nutritional value while reducing the purine content in foods:

Grilling:

Grilling is a low-purine method that imparts a delicious smoky flavor to meats and vegetables without the need for added fats. Opt for lean cuts of meat to keep purine levels in check.

Baking:

Baking allows for a controlled cooking environment, preserving the natural flavors of ingredients. It is a suitable method for proteins like fish, chicken, and tofu, minimizing the need for excessive oils or high-purine ingredients.

Steaming:

Steaming is a gentle cooking technique that retains the texture and nutritional value of foods. It's particularly suitable for vegetables, seafood, and grains, helping to maintain a gout-friendly balance.

Poaching:

Poaching involves cooking food in a simmering liquid, such as broth or water. This method is ideal for delicate proteins like fish and chicken, minimizing the addition of fats or purine-rich ingredients.

Slow Cooking:

Slow cooking at lower temperatures allows flavors to develop over time. It's a convenient method for preparing gout-friendly stews and soups with lean meats, legumes, and vegetables.

Sautéing with Minimal Oil:

Sautéing with a small amount of oil preserves the natural flavors of ingredients while minimizing the addition of excess fats. Choose healthy oils like olive oil for its anti-inflammatory properties.

Stir-Frying:

Stir-frying quickly cooks ingredients in a small amount of oil, making it a suitable option for gout-friendly meals.

Include a variety of colorful vegetables and lean proteins for a balanced dish.

Broiling:

Broiling exposes food to high heat from above, allowing excess fats to drip away. It's a convenient method for cooking lean meats and vegetables with minimal purine release.

Microwaving:

Microwaving is a quick and efficient way to cook foods, especially vegetables, without the need for added fats. It helps to preserve nutrients and reduce the purine content of the dish.

Boiling with Low-Purine Broths:

Boiling foods in low-purine broths or water is a straightforward method that preserves the natural flavors of ingredients while minimizing the intake of purines.

Flavorful Low-Fat Alternatives

Maintaining a low-fat diet is crucial for gout management, but it doesn't mean sacrificing taste. Explore these flavorful low-fat alternatives to enhance the palatability of your meals while adhering to gout-friendly principles:

Herbs and Spices:

Infuse dishes with a variety of herbs and spices such as basil, thyme, rosemary, and cumin to add depth and complexity to flavors without relying on fats.

Citrus Zest:

Utilize the zest of citrus fruits like lemons, limes, and oranges to impart vibrant, zesty notes to dishes, enhancing taste without the need for added fats.

Vinegar and Balsamic Glaze:

Incorporate vinegar and balsamic glaze to add acidity and sweetness to meals. They offer robust flavors without contributing to overall fat content.

Mustard and Horseradish:

Mustard and horseradish are low-calorie condiments that provide a spicy kick, making them excellent choices for enhancing the taste of various dishes.

Low-Fat Broths and Stocks:

Opt for low-fat or fat-free broths and stocks as flavorful bases for soups, stews, and sauces. They add richness without the excess fat content.

Tomato-Based Sauces:

Tomato sauces, whether homemade or store-bought, can serve as a flavorful, low-fat alternative to creamy or buttery sauces. Include herbs and garlic for added taste.

Soy Sauce and Tamari:

Use low-sodium soy sauce or tamari to add a savory, umami flavor to dishes. Be mindful of portion sizes to manage sodium intake.

Greek Yogurt:

Substitute full-fat dairy with plain, non-fat Greek yogurt. It adds creaminess to dishes like dressings and dips without the saturated fat content.

Salsas and Fresh Relishes:

Fresh salsas and relishes made with ingredients like tomatoes, onions, and cilantro can elevate the taste of various dishes while remaining low in fat.

Roasted Garlic:

Roasting garlic enhances its natural sweetness and adds a depth of flavor. Use it in sauces, dressings, or as a topping for vegetables and lean proteins.

Chili Peppers and Hot Sauces:

Spice up your meals with chili peppers or hot sauces to add heat and dimension to your dishes without relying on high-fat ingredients.

Low-Fat Marinades:

Create flavorful marinades using ingredients like herbs, citrus, and vinegar to infuse meats and vegetables with taste before cooking.

Honey and Agave Nectar:

For a touch of sweetness, use natural sweeteners like honey or agave nectar in moderation. They can enhance flavors without adding unnecessary fats.

CHAPTER FOUR

BREAKFAST DELIGHTS

Greek Yogurt Parfait:

Ingredients:

- 1 cup non-fat Greek yogurt
- 1/2 cup fresh berries (e.g., blueberries, strawberries)
- 2 tablespoons granola

Instructions:

- In a glass or bowl, layer Greek yogurt with fresh berries.
- Top with granola for a satisfying crunch.

Vegetable Omelette:

Ingredients:

- 2 eggs, beaten
- 1/4 cup diced bell peppers
- 1/4 cup diced tomatoes
- 1/4 cup spinach leaves
- Salt and pepper to taste

Instructions:

- In a non-stick skillet, sauté vegetables until tender.
- Pour beaten eggs over the veggies, cook until set, and fold for a tasty omelette.

Oatmeal with Fresh Fruit:

Ingredients:

- 1/2 cup old-fashioned oats
- 1 cup water or low-fat milk
- 1/2 banana, sliced
- Handful of sliced almonds

Instructions:

- Cook oats with water or milk, top with banana slices and almonds for added flavor and texture.

Whole Wheat Pancakes:

Ingredients:

- 1 cup whole wheat flour
- 1 tablespoon baking powder
- 1 egg
- 1 cup low-fat milk

Instructions:

Mix ingredients until smooth, cook on a griddle, and serve with fresh fruit.

Smoothie Bowl:

Ingredients:

- 1 cup frozen mixed berries
- 1/2 banana
- 1/2 cup non-fat Greek yogurt
- 1 tablespoon chia seeds

Instructions:

- Blend ingredients until smooth, pour into a bowl, and top with chia seeds for added crunch.

Avocado Toast:

Ingredients:

- 1 slice whole grain bread
- 1/2 ripe avocado, mashed
- Pinch of red pepper flakes
- Salt and pepper to taste

Instructions:

- Toast the bread, spread mashed avocado, and sprinkle with red pepper flakes, salt, and pepper.

Chia Pudding:

Ingredients:

- 2 tablespoons chia seeds

- 1 cup unsweetened almond milk

- 1/2 teaspoon vanilla extract

- Fresh berries for topping

Instructions:

- Mix chia seeds, almond milk, and vanilla extract. Refrigerate overnight and top with fresh berries before serving.

Fruit Salad with Cottage Cheese:

Ingredients:

- 1 cup mixed fresh fruit (e.g., pineapple, melon, berries)

- 1/2 cup low-fat cottage cheese

- Drizzle of honey (optional)

Instructions:

- Combine fresh fruit and cottage cheese, drizzle with honey if desired.

Quinoa Breakfast Bowl:

Ingredients:

- 1/2 cup cooked quinoa

- 1/4 cup sliced almonds

- 1/2 cup sliced peaches

- 1 tablespoon honey

Instructions:

- Mix cooked quinoa with almonds, top with sliced peaches, and drizzle with honey.

Egg and Vegetable Breakfast Wrap:

Ingredients:

- 1 whole wheat tortilla

- 2 eggs, scrambled

- Handful of spinach

- 1/4 cup diced tomatoes

Instructions:

- Fill the tortilla with scrambled eggs, spinach, and tomatoes. Roll it up for a satisfying breakfast wrap.

CHAPTER FIVE

LUNCHTIME FAVORITES

Grilled Chicken Salad:

Ingredients:

- Grilled chicken breast strips
- Mixed salad greens
- Cherry tomatoes
- Cucumber slices
- Balsamic vinaigrette dressing

Instructions:

- Toss grilled chicken strips, salad greens, tomatoes, and cucumbers. Drizzle with balsamic vinaigrette.

Quinoa and Vegetable Stir-Fry:

Ingredients:

- Cooked quinoa
- Mixed vegetables (broccoli, bell peppers, carrots)
- Tofu or shrimp
- Soy sauce
- Sesame oil

Instructions:

- Stir-fry vegetables and protein in sesame oil. Add cooked quinoa and soy sauce, toss until well combined.

Turkey and Avocado Wrap:

Ingredients:

- Sliced turkey breast
- Whole wheat wrap
- Avocado slices
- Lettuce
- Dijon mustard

Instructions:

- Layer turkey, avocado, and lettuce on a wrap. Drizzle with Dijon mustard, roll, and enjoy.

Mediterranean Chickpea Salad:

Ingredients:

- Canned chickpeas (rinsed)
- Cherry tomatoes
- Cucumber, diced
- Feta cheese
- Olive oil and lemon dressing

Instructions:

- Combine chickpeas, tomatoes, cucumber, and feta. Drizzle with olive oil and lemon dressing.

Vegetarian Quiche:

Ingredients:

- Pie crust
- Eggs
- Spinach
- Cherry tomatoes
- Feta cheese

Instructions:

- Whisk eggs, mix in spinach, tomatoes, and feta. Pour into pie crust and bake until set.

Salmon and Asparagus Foil Packets:

Ingredients:

- Salmon fillet
- Asparagus spears
- Lemon slices
- Olive oil
- Garlic, minced

Instructions:

- Place salmon and asparagus on foil. Drizzle with olive oil, add lemon slices and minced garlic. Seal packets and bake.

Caprese Sandwich:

Ingredients:

- Sliced mozzarella
- Tomato slices
- Fresh basil leaves
- Whole grain bread
- Balsamic glaze

Instructions:

- Layer mozzarella, tomatoes, and basil on bread. Drizzle with balsamic glaze and close the sandwich.

Vegetable and Chickpea Curry:

Ingredients:

- Mixed vegetables (zucchini, bell peppers, carrots)
- Chickpeas
- Curry sauce
- Brown rice

Instructions:

- Sauté vegetables, add chickpeas and curry sauce. Serve over cooked brown rice.

Shrimp and Vegetable Skewers:

Ingredients:

- Shrimp
- Bell peppers, onions, cherry tomatoes
- Olive oil
- Lemon juice

Instructions:

- Thread shrimp and veggies onto skewers. Grill or bake, then drizzle with olive oil and lemon juice.

Pesto Pasta with Cherry Tomatoes:

Ingredients:

- Whole wheat pasta
- Pesto sauce
- Cherry tomatoes, halved
- Parmesan cheese

Instructions:

- Cook pasta, toss with pesto, and mix in cherry tomatoes. Sprinkle with Parmesan cheese before serving.

CHAPTER SIX

DINNER OPTIONS

Baked Lemon Herb Chicken:

Ingredients:

- Chicken breasts
- Lemon juice
- Garlic, minced
- Fresh herbs (rosemary, thyme)
- Olive oil

Instructions:

- Marinate chicken in lemon juice, garlic, and herbs. Bake until fully cooked, drizzle with olive oil before serving.

Vegetarian Stuffed Bell Peppers:

Ingredients:

- Bell peppers
- Quinoa
- Black beans
- Corn
- Salsa

Instructions:

- Cook quinoa, mix with black beans, corn, and salsa. Stuff bell peppers, bake until peppers are tender.

Salmon and Asparagus Sheet Pan Dinner:

Ingredients:

- Salmon fillets
- Asparagus spears
- Potatoes, sliced
- Lemon slices
- Olive oil

Instructions:

- Arrange salmon, asparagus, and potatoes on a sheet pan. Drizzle with olive oil, add lemon slices. Roast until cooked.

Vegetable and Lentil Curry:

Ingredients:

- Lentils
- Mixed vegetables (cauliflower, peas, carrots)
- Coconut milk
- Curry spices

Instructions:

- Cook lentils, add mixed vegetables, coconut milk, and curry spices. Simmer until vegetables are tender.

Grilled Eggplant and Tomato Stack:

Ingredients:

- Eggplant slices
- Tomato slices
- Mozzarella cheese
- Basil leaves
- Balsamic glaze

Instructions:

- Grill eggplant slices, layer with tomatoes, mozzarella, and basil. Drizzle with balsamic glaze.

Turkey and Vegetable Stir-Fry:

Ingredients:

- Ground turkey
- Mixed stir-fry vegetables
- Soy sauce
- Ginger, minced
- Brown rice

Instructions:

- Stir-fry turkey and vegetables in soy sauce and ginger. Serve over cooked brown rice.

Cauliflower and Chickpea Curry:

Ingredients:

- Cauliflower florets
- Chickpeas
- Curry sauce
- Spinach

Instructions:

- Cook cauliflower and chickpeas in curry sauce. Add spinach and simmer until wilted.

Mushroom and Spinach Stuffed Chicken Breast:

Ingredients:

- Chicken breasts
- Mushrooms, chopped
- Spinach
- Garlic, minced
- Mozzarella cheese

Instructions:

- Sauté mushrooms, spinach, and garlic. Stuff chicken breasts, top with mozzarella, and bake until done.

Whole Grain Pasta Primavera:

Ingredients:

- Whole grain pasta
- Assorted vegetables (bell peppers, cherry tomatoes, broccoli)
- Olive oil
- Parmesan cheese

Instructions:

- Cook pasta, toss with sautéed vegetables, olive oil, and Parmesan cheese.

Teriyaki Tofu and Vegetable Skewers:

Ingredients:

- Tofu, cubed
- Bell peppers, onions, zucchini
- Teriyaki sauce
- Brown rice

Instructions:

- Marinate tofu and vegetables in teriyaki sauce. Skewer and grill until veggies are tender. Serve over brown rice.

43

CHAPTER SEVEN

SATISFYING SNACKS

Greek Yogurt Parfait:

Ingredients:

- Greek yogurt
- Fresh berries
- Granola

Instructions:

- In a glass or bowl, layer Greek yogurt with fresh berries and granola for a satisfying and nutritious snack.

Hummus and Veggie Sticks:

Ingredients:

- Hummus
- Carrot sticks, cucumber slices, bell pepper strips

Instructions:

- Dip assorted vegetable sticks into hummus for a crunchy and flavorful snack.

Apple Slices with Almond Butter:

Ingredients:

- Apple slices
- Almond butter

Instructions:

- Spread almond butter on apple slices for a delicious combination of sweetness and nuttiness.

Hard-Boiled Eggs with Avocado:

Ingredients:

- Hard-boiled eggs
- Avocado, sliced

Instructions:

- Slice hard-boiled eggs and top with avocado slices for a protein-packed and satisfying snack.

Trail Mix with Nuts and Dried Fruit:

Ingredients:

- Mixed nuts (almonds, walnuts, cashews)
- Dried fruit (raisins, cranberries)
- Dark chocolate chips

Instructions:

- Mix nuts, dried fruit, and dark chocolate chips for a portable and energizing snack.

Cottage Cheese with Pineapple:

Ingredients:

- Low-fat cottage cheese
- Pineapple chunks

Instructions:

- Combine cottage cheese with pineapple chunks for a sweet and creamy snack.

Rice Cakes with Peanut Butter and Banana:

Ingredients:

- Rice cakes
- Peanut butter
- Banana slices

Instructions:

- Spread peanut butter on rice cakes and top with banana slices for a satisfying and crunchy treat.

Vegetable Sushi Rolls:

Ingredients:

- Nori sheets

- Brown rice

- Avocado, cucumber, carrot

- Soy sauce for dipping

Instructions:

- Roll brown rice and sliced vegetables in nori sheets for a homemade vegetable sushi snack.

Edamame with Sea Salt:

Ingredients:

- Edamame (steamed or boiled)

- Sea salt

Instructions:

- Sprinkle steamed or boiled edamame with sea salt for a simple and protein-rich snack.

Cherry Tomatoes with Mozzarella:

Ingredients:

- Cherry tomatoes

- Mozzarella cheese balls

- Basil leaves

- Balsamic glaze (optional)

Instructions:

- Skewer cherry tomatoes, mozzarella balls, and basil leaves for a tasty caprese-inspired snack. Drizzle with balsamic glaze if desired.

CHAPTER EIGHT

DESSERTS WITHOUT REGRET

Mixed Berry Parfait:

Ingredients:

- Mixed berries (strawberries, blueberries, raspberries)
- Greek yogurt
- Granola

Instructions:

- In a glass, layer Greek yogurt with mixed berries and granola for a guilt-free parfait.

Dark Chocolate-Dipped Strawberries:

Ingredients:

- Fresh strawberries
- Dark chocolate (70% cocoa or higher)

Instructions:

- Melt dark chocolate, dip strawberries, and place on parchment paper to cool for a decadent treat.

Chia Seed Pudding:

Ingredients:

- Chia seeds
- Almond milk
- Vanilla extract
- Fresh fruit for topping

Instructions:

- Mix chia seeds, almond milk, and vanilla extract. Refrigerate until it thickens, then top with fresh fruit.

Frozen Banana Bites:

Ingredients:

- Bananas, sliced
- Almond butter
- Dark chocolate, melted

Instructions:

- Spread almond butter between banana slices, dip in melted dark chocolate, and freeze for a delightful bite.

Yogurt and Berry Ice Pops:

Ingredients:

- Greek yogurt
- Mixed berries

- Honey

Instructions:

Blend Greek yogurt, berries, and honey. Pour into popsicle molds and freeze for a refreshing treat.

Baked Apple with Cinnamon:

Ingredients:

- Apple, cored and sliced
- Cinnamon
- Walnuts (optional)

Instructions:

- Sprinkle apple slices with cinnamon, bake until tender, and top with chopped walnuts if desired.

Coconut Mango Sorbet:

Ingredients:

- Frozen mango chunks
- Coconut milk
- Lime juice

Instructions:

- Blend frozen mango, coconut milk, and lime juice until smooth. Freeze for a tropical sorbet.

Protein-Packed Chocolate Mousse:

Ingredients:

- Silken tofu
- Dark chocolate
- Maple syrup

Instructions:

- Blend silken tofu, melted dark chocolate, and maple syrup until creamy. Chill before serving.

Baked Cinnamon Bananas:

Ingredients:

- Bananas
- Cinnamon
- Honey

Instructions:

- Slice bananas, sprinkle with cinnamon, drizzle with honey, and bake until golden for a warm dessert.

Almond Flour Blueberry Muffins:

Ingredients:

- Almond flour
- Eggs

- Baking powder

- Blueberries

Instructions:

- Mix almond flour, eggs, and baking powder. Fold in blueberries and bake for a grain-free muffin option.

Water:

Description: The cornerstone of hydration, water helps flush out uric acid and prevent kidney stones.

How to Enjoy: Drink plain or infuse with slices of cucumber, lemon, or mint for added flavor.

Herbal Teas:

Description: Herbal teas like chamomile, ginger, and peppermint are naturally caffeine-free and can contribute to hydration.

How to Enjoy: Steep herbal tea bags in hot water and enjoy plain or with a touch of honey.

Cherry Juice:

Description: Tart cherry juice may have anti-inflammatory properties and has been associated with lower levels of uric acid.

How to Enjoy: Drink a small glass of pure, unsweetened cherry juice or dilute with water.

Green Tea:

Description: Green tea contains antioxidants and may have anti-inflammatory effects, potentially beneficial for gout.

How to Enjoy: Brew green tea and enjoy it hot or cold. Add a slice of lemon for extra flavor.

Low-Fat Milk:

Description: Low-fat or fat-free milk is a good source of calcium and may help lower the risk of gout attacks.

How to Enjoy: Drink a glass of milk or use it in smoothies and beverages.

Vegetable Juice:

Description: Freshly squeezed vegetable juices, especially those with celery and leafy greens, can be hydrating and nutritious.

How to Enjoy: Juice vegetables like celery, cucumber, and spinach for a refreshing beverage.

Water with Lemon:

Description: Lemon may help alkalize the body and reduce acidity, potentially benefiting gout management.

How to Enjoy: Squeeze fresh lemon juice into water for a simple, hydrating drink.

Coconut Water:

Description: Coconut water is a natural electrolyte-rich beverage that can contribute to hydration.

How to Enjoy: Drink coconut water on its own or use it as a base for smoothies.

Filtered Alkaline Water:

Description: Some evidence suggests that maintaining a slightly alkaline pH may be beneficial for gout.

How to Enjoy: Choose filtered water with a pH slightly above 7 for regular hydration.

Ginger Infused Water:

Description: Ginger has anti-inflammatory properties and can add a flavorful twist to plain water.

How to Enjoy: Infuse water with fresh ginger slices for a refreshing and potentially soothing beverage.

CONCLUSION

In conclusion, managing gout through dietary choices involves a thoughtful and balanced approach. Understanding the impact of certain foods and adopting a gout-friendly diet can contribute significantly to reducing the frequency and severity of gout attacks. Key considerations include avoiding high-purine foods, moderating intake of purine-containing proteins, and staying hydrated with gout-friendly beverages.

The journey to gout management begins with a solid foundation of knowledge about the condition. Recognizing the importance of maintaining a healthy weight, staying physically active, and making mindful dietary choices can contribute to overall well-being and reduce the risk of gout flares.

Our exploration covered various aspects, from understanding gout and the significance of a gout-friendly diet to practical guidelines for meal planning. We delved into specific topics such as identifying foods to avoid, incorporating low-purine cooking methods, and embracing flavorful, low-fat alternatives. We also explored smart ingredient substitutions and provided a variety of delightful and satisfying recipes for breakfast, lunch, dinner, and snacks that align with gout management principles.

It's essential to note that individual responses to dietary changes may vary, and consulting with healthcare professionals or registered dietitians is crucial for personalized advice tailored to specific health conditions and needs. The gout-friendly recommendations discussed aim to strike a balance between flavor, nutrition, and gout management, promoting a sustainable and enjoyable approach to a healthier lifestyle.

By incorporating the insights and practical tips discussed, individuals can take proactive steps towards managing gout, fostering overall well-being, and enjoying a varied and delicious array of foods that align with gout-friendly principles.

www.ingramcontent.com/pod-product-compliance
Lightning Source LLC
Chambersburg PA
CBHW071107260726
48661CB00006B/2520